The A-to-Z Guide for New Mothers

JAYNE GARRISON

POCKET GUIDES
Tyndale House Publishers, Inc.
Wheaton, Illinois

Acknowledgments
Chess, Stella, "Are You Jealous of Your Children Without Knowing It?" *Family Circle*, November 1976.

Spock, Benjamin, *Baby and Child Care*, Simon and Schuster, New York, 1974.

Scripture quotations are from the King James Version of *The Holy Bible*, except for those marked *TLB*, which are from *The Living Bible*.

The information presented in this book is based on personal experience and opinion. Advice about medical and dietary matters should be checked out with your physician or your baby's pediatrician.

Adapted from *The ABC's of Christian Mothering* by Jayne Garrison
© 1979 by Jayne Garrison, published by Tyndale House Publishers, Inc.

First printing, October 1986
Library of Congress Catalog Card Number 86-50594
ISBN 0-8423-0008-2
© 1986 by Jayne Garrison
All rights reserved
Printed in the United States of America

Contents

Introduction: What Is a Mother? 7

A
Appearance—
a more attractive you 9

B
Baby-sitters—
finding and keeping them 13

C
Colic—those terrible tears 17

D
Dads—tapping their potential . . . 21

E
Everyday Things—
baths, diapers, beds, and toys . . . 24

F
Food Time—feeding Baby 31

G
Games—simple fun with Baby . . . 35

H
Housekeeping—
hints to banish chaos 37

I
Illness—coping with the nasties . . 42

J
Jealousy—harnessing the lion . . . 46

K
Keepsakes—
going down memory lane 48

L
Layette—what Baby will wear . . . 51

M
Mothering—the gentle art 53

N
Natural Ways—
childbirth and nursing 56

O
Overweight—
what goes on must come off 62

P
Pacifiers—solving the dilemma . . . 65

Q
Quiet Time—
moments for your baby and you . . 67

R
Romance—restoring the sparkle . . 70

S
Schedules—getting yours in order . 73

T
Traveling—have Baby, will bundle . 76

U
Unity—plugging for each other . . . 79

V
Vaccinations—
keeping up with Baby's health . . . 81

W
Working—pros and cons 83

X
X's of Family Fun—
the secret's out 86

Y
Yes and No—
discipline with love 88

Z
Zzzzz—
sounds with meaning 91

Other Books for New Mothers 95

INTRODUCTION

What Is a Mother?

Congratulations! You are a mother, the most important person in the world to that tiny bundle of perfection you carried home from the hospital.

Motherhood holds many choices. You can be respected like a good boss, or you can be feared like a mighty tyrant. You can cling possessively to your child until he becomes a social cripple, or you can let go daily as he broadens his boundaries.

How will you know which direction to turn? By adopting an attitude of trust in God, by seeking the support of family and friends, and by following the guidance of books like this one!

A baby is an inestimable burden and blessing.
—Mark Twain

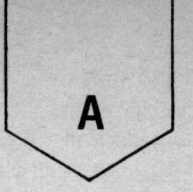

Appearance— a more attractive you

During the first few weeks of motherhood, the simplest toiletry may seem an impossible feat. So, why not try the following suggestions for quick inspiration?

EVERYDAY PRIORITIES
As a mother, you deserve the same care that you gave yourself as a mother-to-be:

You need:

- a balanced diet
- plenty of sleep
- fresh air
- correction of physical disorders
- exercise

Beyond these basics, however, there are certain areas to which every well-groomed mother should give special attention.

SKIN CARE BASICS
Dry skin. Because of all the hormonal changes taking place in your body, motherhood is apt to leave your skin drier than usual. To relieve dry skin, try taking a daily oil bath, or follow your shower with a generous anointing of body lotion.

Chapped hands. Now your hands are constantly in and out of water, rinsing diapers, preparing formula, or just keeping things clean. Station a bottle of hand cream beside each sink, and use it.

Stretch marks. Often called the badge of motherhood, striae never entirely disappear, but you can minimize them with the daily application of a cream or lotion designed for this purpose.

Complexion. Again due to hormone imbalance, your complexion may be temporarily dry or oily after the birth of a baby. Cosmetics that were once just right may no longer be suitable. When this happens, ask a beauty consultant to help you select the appropriate cleansing and moisturizing products.

HAIR CARE
Style. Because there's no time for daily hairwashing, a short blow-dry cut may save your day. If you're reluctant to part with those long tresses, perhaps a ponytail tied with a colorful ribbon would solve your new hair

problem. Keep a bag of tricks up your sleeve —dry shampoo, an inexpensive wig, a collection of pretty scarves.

Falling hair. It's not uncommon for women to notice a large hair loss after pregnancy. Usually the hair resumes its normal growth pattern in a few months. But if this condition should cause you worry, consult your doctor.

Hair breakage. This, too, is a frequent complaint of new mothers. To remedy the situation, give yourself a hot oil treatment once a week or use one of the many instant treatments now available on the market. It might be wise to skip those nightly brushings, and to avoid the use of hair rollers whenever possible.

Homemade oil treatment. Apply one tablespoon of olive oil or castor oil to your scalp with a cotton ball. Massage into the scalp. Wrap your head in a hot towel, and then step into a hot steamy bath or shower.

DENTAL HYGIENE

Keep up with your daily brushings and yearly dental checkup. If you neglect your teeth now, chances are you'll be in line for extensive repair work about the same time that Junior needs braces.

FRAGRANCE

Use fragrance every day. There are three important reasons to smell pleasant—Baby, Hubby, and you.

EXTRA HINTS

The beauty box. Sharing a bathroom with the family? Avoid the frustration of hunting for toiletries by preparing a beauty box to keep in the bedroom. This can be nothing more than a shoe box in which you keep a comb and brush, a razor, body lotion, deodorant, and simple makeup basics.

Sore muscle reliever. Stand under a shower as hot as you can tolerate for about five minutes, or add a half cup of Epsom salt to the bath water.

For quick energy. Take an alternatingly hot and cold shower.

To cool off. Bathe in slightly cool, not cold, water. Dust yourself with bath powder.

Wardrobe saver. Keep your clothing fresh all day by wearing a smock when feeding or bathing Baby. (One of Hubby's old shirts will do nicely.)

B

*Baby-sitters—
finding and keeping them*

Parents seeking a good baby-sitter usually rely upon the daughters of well-thought-of neighbors, recommendations from other parents, and sometimes referrals from a church secretary who knows her congregation.

GETTING ACQUAINTED
One friend of mine always invites a new baby-sitter over for a get-acquainted session before she actually hires her. "Could you come over for about thirty minutes to meet my children and see if you might be interested in baby-sitting?" is the way she tactfully puts it.

This is a marvelous chance to observe not only the maturity of the girl, but her speech, mode of dress, and attitude toward children.

After you've chosen your baby-sitter, perhaps the first time you'd like her to sit for you is during the day for an hour or two. Arrange transportation details, then ask her to be available about twenty minutes early so that you can show her around the house and still have time to leave proper instructions.

SETTING GUIDELINES

As you show her through the house, be clear as to which rooms she and the children may have access to. If guard gates are providing safety boundaries for small children, emphasize their purpose. Point out the heater and air-conditioner controls, and explain how to regulate the room temperature. It's generally assumed that the baby-sitter may watch television or listen to the stereo, so save yourself a repair bill and show her how this equipment works.

A baby-sitter should never be left to guess certain things about your child. For instance, let the baby-sitter know each child's toilet procedure, in writing if necessary.

Don't forget to tell the baby-sitter about those all-important bedtime comforts such as special blankets, toys, night-lights, and window shades. Show her where to find diapers and fresh clothing, but *never* ask the baby-sitter to give baths—a dangerous responsibility for her. Instead, have your children dressed and ready for bed before you leave for the evening.

Be sure to leave a hearty snack on a tray for the baby-sitter.

What about extra duties? You may have to ask her to feed the children once in a while, but it's important to remember that any additional work will only keep her away from her first duty—the children.

Before saying "good-bye," review the rules of the house. It's perfectly all right to insist upon no telephone chats and no visitors. Place the Baby-sitter Information Chart (page 16) next to the telephone.

One good way to insure that your rules are followed is to warn the baby-sitter that although you plan to be home at a given time, you might call or even return unexpectedly. If you come home to find your children asleep or playing happily, your house in the order you left it, and the baby-sitter quietly reading or watching television, you've found yourself a gem. Give her the respect of always returning on time, pay her promptly and fairly, and compliment her on a job well done. But if your children are unhappy, your home is dismantled, and there are telltale signs of broken rules, this person is not for you.

Baby-sitters are never as scarce as they sometimes seem to be. Co-ops, professional baby-sitters, and child care centers can be found in almost every community. And don't neglect grandmothers and aunties!

BABY-SITTER INFORMATION CHART

We, _____,
     (your name)
will be at _____
          (your location)
Their phone number is _____.
We will return home at _____.
Our address here is _____.
Our phone number here is _____.
You are baby-sitting _____, age ____.
                    _____, age ____.
                    _____, age ____.
                    _____, age ____.

EMERGENCY/POLICE NUMBER: _____.
Our Pediatrician is Dr. _____
at _____
     (phone number)

SPECIAL THINGS TO REMEMBER:
(1) *Type of snack* to give: _____
                             (describe)
                        at _____
                                (time)
(2) *Bedtime* is at _____
                 (time)
(3) *Bedtime rituals* are _____
_____

PHONE MESSAGES:

C

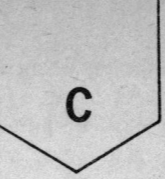

Colic—those terrible tears

A hard, persistent cry accompanied by the drawing up of legs and a distended abdomen fits the baby book's description of colic to a tee. Some babies pass a great deal of gas and seem to have these spells of crying only at a certain time of the day.

Other babies cry either with colic or just plain irritableness from morning till night, and these little critters can really baffle us parents.

WHAT CAUSES COLIC?
Some experts say that colic often occurs in babies with a family history of eczema, hay fever, asthma, or other allergic disorders. So some mothers, thinking their baby is allergic to cow's milk, take this as a cue to begin a three-month regimen of formula switching.

And then there's the theory that colic is brought upon by nervous mothers. While it's true that most mothers with colicky babies are nervous, let's be honest—who wouldn't be nervous after listening to the cry of a helpless infant for hours on end?

Finally, the most frequently given reason for colic today is an immature digestive system. This may not mean much to you and me, but it goes a long way when Grandma or the nosy neighbor wants to know what's wrong with your baby.

TEN WAYS TO ALLEVIATE COLIC

Dr. Benjamin Spock reminds us that colic lasts about three months, is fairly common, and doesn't seem to do the baby any harm. "On the contrary," he says, "it occurs most often in babies that are developing and growing well." Great. But in the meantime, your baby is crying—what can you do about that?

1. *If you suspect that your baby has colic, first get in touch with your doctor.* He may be able to give your baby relief with a mild medication.
2. *Develop a mental checklist.* Is your baby hungry? Wet? Cold? Lonely? Sleepy? Just plain fretful?
3. *Give the baby his medication, play with him for a few minutes, and then lay him on his tummy in his bed.* Babies with colic are usually more comfortable on their stomachs, and this procedure often works best for helping the baby fall asleep. But if your baby stops crying only when you're holding him, by all means, hold him. You'll both feel happier.

4. *In between medication dosages, try a pacifier, walking, rocking, riding in the car, or a warm hot water bottle placed on the baby's tummy.* Please do check the heat of the bottle, making sure that you can comfortably rest it against your wrist, and wrap it in a diaper.
5. *Offer frequent, small feedings.* Do this instead of trying to stick to a schedule, always remembering to burp Baby afterward.
6. *If your baby seems to be at his worst when you leave the house, avoid large crowds and drafty places.* Some mothers have found that in extreme cases of colic it works best not to even take the baby outside for as long as the colic persists.
7. *Keep the baby always comfortably warm.* Some colicky babies like to be swaddled in receiving blankets most of the time.
8. *Arrange with your husband to take turns napping during those most difficult hours at the end of an exhausting day.*
9. *Never give the baby any medication not prescribed for him by your doctor.*
10. *Make an effort to relax.* Put the relaxation exercises that you learned in your childbirth classes into practice again, fix yourself a refreshing beverage, and rest your feet.

WHAT IF YOU'RE NURSING?
Both bottle- and breast-fed infants can have colic, but if you're nursing, you deserve spe-

cial encouragement. A colicky baby doesn't always sleep well, and you're going to feel tired and run-down. In order to get as much rest as possible, try to curtail all but the most basic activities.

If household help is out of the question, let the house go, knowing that in a few months there'll be more than enough time to scrub and clean.

Above all, don't quit nursing just because of colic. Your baby needs the warmth of your arms, the smell of your body. You can benefit from the calm that comes with the letdown of milk. Fortunately, you should have plenty of milk because colicky babies are enthusiastic nursers.

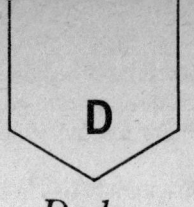

Dads—
tapping their potential

Like mothering, fathering doesn't necessarily come naturally. But while women can pick up trade secrets from friends, relatives, and books written especially for them, men have few resources to turn to. That's where you, the mother, can help.

B.B.—BEFORE BABY
Begin to prepare together:

1. Entertain.
2. Go out as often as you feel up to it.
3. Sleep late on Saturdays.
4. Begin gradually breaking away from the idea of a twosome world.
5. Decide together when you'll announce your pregnancy, what you'll name the baby, where the baby will be born, and where he'll sleep once he's home.
6. Walk together each day, and let your thoughts wander toward the future.
7. Talk about the layette, the nursery, and all the baby equipment you'll need.

8. When its time to shop, go together, browsing through garage sales and antique shops for that one truly unique item.
9. Place child care books in strategic spots around the house.
10. Attend not only childbirth education classes, but baby care classes as well.
11. Plan on a cooperative delivery with Dad not just present, but helping. And top it all off with "rooming-in." This provides a wonderful opportunity for breaking a father into diapering and feeding.

A.B.—AFTER BABY
Encourage fatherly feelings:

1. Together you can bathe the baby before bedtime and rock him during those spurts of wakefulness.
2. Be patient—Dad is sure to fit into the fathering mold sometime during the first year.
3. Arrange for your husband to entertain the baby while you bathe each night.
4. Start the custom of father and child dinners. Dad feeds the baby while drinking a glass of iced tea and munching on cheese. Where are *you?* Fixing dinner, of course.
5. Plan for your husband to bathe the baby once a week.
6. Whenever possible, let Dad accompany

you, or go in your place, on your baby's visits to the doctor.
7. Let your husband select and purchase some of the baby's clothing.
8. Encourage a quiet time between father and child before bedtime. This can begin with rocking and grow into bedtime reading.

As you watch your husband and child become friends, you'll notice that even a baby senses the specialness of Dad. With such rapport, is it any wonder that a baby's first word is usually "Da-Da"?

Finally, remember that your child is an extension of you—your gift to your husband. His total acceptance and absolute love for your gift is one of the many ways of saying, "I love you." And isn't that what being a parent is all about anyway?

E

Everyday Things— baths, diapers, beds, and toys

BATHING

It's normal to feel shaky about your baby's first bath. The following steps will help you prepare for it.

Equipment. Store the baby's bath needs all together in a pretty wicker basket decorated with ribbons, an ordinary utility tray, or anything that has a handle and can be easily carried from nursery to bathing area. The bath basket should contain:

- a bar of mild soap and soap dish
- cotton balls and swabs
- baby oil, lotion, and powder
- a soft washcloth, towel, and extra diaper pins.

Where. Choose a warm, quiet spot for the bath. The kitchen table or bathroom vanity is usually a wise choice.

When. Bathe the baby at the same time each day—he'll soon learn to expect and enjoy his bath. Pick whatever time suits you best, but don't bathe him right after a feeding. He needs a quiet time to follow his meals.

It's a good idea to take the phone off the hook during the baby's bath time. If it's really important, the caller will try again.

The sponge bath. Your doctor will probably recommend a sponge bath for your baby until the navel or the circumcision is healed. For this, you can either hold the baby in your lap or lay him on a soft towel on the table where you have already placed the bath basket, clean clothing, and a small bowl of water around 95°-100° F. (this will feel comfortable to your elbow). Now you're set.

1. Gently clean outer nose and *outer* ears with cotton swabs.
2. Clean face with a cotton ball dipped in warm water.
3. Shampoo scalp three times a week and oil head daily. To rinse, hold Baby's head (face up) and back over a basin of water. Pat dry.
4. Remove shirt. Soap his chest, arms, and hands, paying attention to folds and creases of skin. Rinse with warm water and pat dry. Turn Baby over; soap the back and buttocks. Rinse with warm water. Pat dry. Return Baby to his back and cover the chest with a towel.

The tub bath. When the baby is around three months old, it's a good time to start the tub bath. Using a small plastic tub with a towel placed on the bottom to prevent slipping is one of the best ways to bathe an infant. Aside from putting Baby into water, there's really not much difference between a sponge bath and a tub bath.

1. Shampoo hair first. To rinse, hold Baby over tub in the crook of your arm. Dry hair before continuing bath.
2. Clean nose with cotton swabs, face and ears with soft washcloth.
3. Undress Baby and place him in the tub with one arm around him, supporting him at all times. Hold on to the outer arm for greater security.
4. Soap Baby, rinse, and wrap him immediately in a towel. Pat dry. Powder and dress him. Continue to use the plastic tub bath until Baby is sitting up well. Then you might like to switch to the kitchen sink and gradually move on to the big bathtub as the baby shows readiness.

Keep Baby's bathtub toys all together in a fishnet shopping bag, and hang it over the shower nozzle.

DIAPERING

Diapering a baby is almost like combing your hair—everyone has her own style. To get an idea of the choices available to you, read the following facts, then take a quick survey through community shops to compare quality and price.

Laundered diapers. Many people suggest

buying three dozen for a starter. Those using coin-operated washing machines, however, will probably enjoy the security of an extra dozen.

A wide choice of diapers awaits you. You'll find gauze, cotton flannel, stretch cotton, and bird's-eye for texture; square, rectangular, prefolded, and snap-ons for style; and newborn, large, and extra large for size. Gauze dries quickly; rectangular ones can be folded in many different ways; and large sizes can be adjusted to fit any size baby.

Diaper service. If you live in an apartment, you'll seriously want to consider diaper service. It will save you so much time and worry that even those parents with washing machines may consider it worthwhile.

Disposables. Once again, we're up against a variety of styles and qualities. Disposables are wonderful, especially for night-time use, for they keep Baby drier than cloth and cut down on that ammonia smell that greets you each morning.

HINTS FOR USING DISPOSABLES
1. Buy good quality diapers to help prevent diaper rash. The less expensive brands are seldom very absorbent, which simply means you'll be changing Baby more often—making it all come out the same financially.
2. Avoid diaper pail odor by discarding disposable diapers in a plastic bag with a twist tie.

3. When Baby's wiggles cause you to damage stick-on tape tabs, secure diaper with an ordinary diaper pin or masking tape.
4. Save on plumbing expenses by emptying diaper in toilet and discarding in the trash.

THE FINE ART OF DIAPER CHANGING
1. Simply fold the soiled portion of the diaper under, as you unpin.
2. Place a waterproof pad under the baby to minimize mess.
3. If he is only wet, there's no need to wash him.
4. After a bowel movement, you should wash the baby's bottom with cotton and water or one of the baby products designed for this purpose.
5. Slip the clean diaper under the baby immediately, and bring it up between the legs.
6. Pin on each side, back overlapping front, being careful to keep a finger between Baby and diaper to avoid pin pricks.
7. Retain diaper pins' sharpness by sticking them into a cake of soap.
8. Keep clean diapers unfolded in a large hamper. The type intended for the use of dirty clothes is excellent. Then, fold as you go.

Note: The older baby will need fewer changes, but continue to let odor and skin condition be your guide.

BEDDING
1. *Purchase a new crib for Baby if possible.* Be aware that secondhand furniture could be painted with leftover paint that may contain lead or may be on its last slat.
2. *Select a good firm mattress.* If you own a washing machine, you might want to pro-

tect the mattress with a thick quilted cover to add comfort and warmth for Baby. Apartment dwellers may find a plastic cover that zips on and off more practical. When Baby soils the sheet, you need only to drop it in your diaper pail and wipe the plastic cover clean.
3. *Add a pillow when Baby is about a year old.* Remember to remove it during bouts of sickness, though, or be sure to wash it extra!

TO SLEEP—PERCHANCE TO DREAM

The young child is sometimes an erratic sleeper—going to bed as late as nine and waking for several hours of play at midnight. Since this can go on for some time, try moving Baby's bedtime up by fifteen minutes every week until you've reached a satisfactory time. Allow him to cry for a good twenty minutes, but no more—crying beyond this may well indicate that the baby needs your attention. He may have gas, or a wet or soiled diaper, for example, or he may be coming down with a bug.

While your baby is learning to sleep through the night, he may call out to you several times, and you can answer his cries with a short nursing, a glass of milk, or a pat on the back. Daddies sometimes have a magic touch with fretful sleepers.

Even after you've got bedtime all worked out, Baby may revert to his old habits now and then. He may have had a bad dream, be teething, or be upset about something that happened during the day. Feel free to pick him up, rock him, or even carry him out to the center of family life.

TOYS

Children need toys to help them learn how to use their bodies and how to live in our world. Toys can add spice to their lives.

As soon as Baby begins to reach for objects, you can begin raiding the house for suitable playthings that will sustain his interest well into his first year—pots and pans, a stack of plastic drinking cups, short-handled wooden spoons, an extra handbag.

Your only boundary is safety. Some household objects may have sharp points, be painted with questionable paint, or be so small that they are easily swallowed and should never be given to a small child.

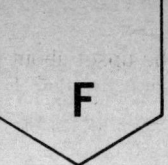

Food Time—feeding Baby

Interest in nutrition heightens during our pregnancy. Later, as we watch our baby grow and develop, we really begin to think twice about food value, especially if we're nursing. When Baby's old enough to start solid food (check with your pediatrician on this), Mother almost collapses from frustration if Baby doesn't eat. Why? Because it is pretty awesome to be totally responsible for somebody else's nutritional well-being.

DECIDING HOW TO FEED BABY
It might be worth noting that nursing mothers seldom have feeding problems. It's not that breast-fed babies are such terrific eaters—it's just that these mothers don't worry about their babies' occasional refusal to eat. They know that Baby is getting his best nutrition from Mother.

Then, too, breast-fed babies thrive on mother's milk for a good five months before graduating to mashed table foods, thus eliminating the intermediate step of bland-tasting commercial baby foods.

On the other hand, bottle babies shouldn't become the victims of nagging, coaxing, or scolding just because they need the nutrients that solid foods offer at an earlier age. Eating is one of nature's pleasures and should be a pleasant experience even for the very young.

> Babies under the age of nine months don't need or care anything about table salt. They get salt naturally from their milk and from some of the foods they eat.

THE FAST AND FABULOUS FOOD MILL

In order for Baby to eat from the family table, you'll need a food mill for grinding his food to an easy-to-eat consistency. After grinding the food in the food mill, soften it with a little breast milk or formula. Follow the doctor's instructions as to order of introduction, and plan your baby's meals from the food list below.

FRUITS

Bananas. An excellent first food, these can be mashed and softened with milk.

Apples. Can be cooked and run through a food mill for the young baby, or peeled and cut into finger slices for the older baby.

Juices. Your doctor will advise you on the use of orange, pineapple, and prune juice.

If you don't plan on making your own, be sure to check the labels on juice bottles and stay away from sugar drinks.

Pears and peaches. The older baby will enjoy these fruits peeled and cut into finger slices.

Oranges and grapefruit. The older baby can also eat small segments of these fruits from which you've removed the seeds.

Other fruits. Some fruits are too tart by themselves for Baby. This is one reason that sugar is often added to commercial baby food fruits. Be your own judge.

EGGS

Because egg white can cause allergy, wait for your doctor's signal before including this part of the egg. In the meantime, hard boil Baby's egg so that the yolk can be easily separated from the white. Mashed with a little milk, egg yolk is often recommended by doctors as an early food.

VEGETABLES

Sweet potatoes. Another good early food, baked sweet potatoes can be mashed and softened with milk. White potato can be prepared in the same manner.

Carrots, squash, beets, asparagus, spinach, broccoli, green beans, and other easy-to-eat vegetables. Simply cook these vegetables in a small amount of water until tender, grind in your food mill, and soften with liquid. Older babies prefer their vegetables served as finger foods.

MEATS
Organ meats. These are good for the very young because they're so high in nutrition and of an easy-to-eat consistency. Beef and chicken liver, chicken gizzards, lamb or veal kidneys, brains, and sweetbreads can be braised or sautéed. Then run them through your food mill and soften with liquid.

Other meats. Fresh or frozen fish, chicken, ham, beef, veal, lamb, and turkey can also be braised or sautéed, ground in your food mill, and softened with liquid. Avoid roast or chops until Baby is well on his way to eating "grown-up" food.

APPETITE PROBLEMS
There will, no doubt, be days when nothing appeals to your baby's palate. This is when you'll cheerfully remove his food and try again later in the day. Perhaps he's teething, coming down with a cold, or just plain not in the mood.

If Baby is more than nine months old, he may be protesting for something a little tastier than high chair fare. Now you may want to add a dash of salt or a speck of catsup.

Mealtime is an opportunity to enjoy savory food, and an opportunity to savor family love.

G

Games—
simple fun with Baby

For a good year or two, you can get by in the doctor's office or airport lounge with a few quiet-time games. Try to remember how your own mother entertained your younger brothers and sisters—the same tricks still work. Here are a few!

FINGER PUPPETS
A fist here and a finger there will turn the most ordinary hand into a delightful puppet. Use your imagination to come up with rabbits, deer, giraffes, and more. If you like, a face can be drawn on your hand with washable ink.

PAT-A-CAKE
One of the most popular and oldest of games, this little rhyme never fails to amuse a baby. Be sure to pat, roll, and make the imaginary B with both your hands and Baby's for these actions teach coordination as well as entertain.

Pat-a-cake, pat-a-cake, Baker's man.
Bake me a cake as fast as you can.
Pat it, and roll it, and mark it with a B,
And put it in the oven for Baby and me.

RIDE LITTLE HORSEY
Cross your legs at the knees. Slowly bounce Baby on your ankle and at the end of the rhyme, gently slide him to the floor.

Ride little horsey,
Ride to town,
Better watch out or
You'll fall down.

Housekeeping—
hints to banish chaos

THE BEDROOM
A comfortable, well-organized bedroom is a must for the new mother. Certainly, you'll clean out drawers and closets before the baby arrives, but don't forget to put away dust collectors. Simplicity will help keep things neater.

The rocker. Most rockers are chosen with just about as much care as a house. You'll spend enough time in this piece of furniture to make the investment of cushions worthwhile. And if the budget allows, it's nice to have a rocker in both the nursery and your bedroom.

Small items. It's a special luxury to have a *television set* in your bedroom, but even a radio will provide a lot of entertainment. Don't forget a *wastepaper basket* beside your bed and a *night-light* for those two o'clock feedings.

Some mothers like to keep a large cardboard box in one corner of the room so that when bric-a-brac becomes overwhelming, everything can be swept quickly in the box and out of sight. (You can do the sorting later when there's more time.)

THE KITCHEN

The state of your kitchen during your postpartum days is of prime importance. The following suggestions can help you get a better handle on organizing it before Baby arrives.

1. Keep things that you use most often on the shelves that are easiest to reach.
2. Eliminate clutter by clearing off an entire shelf just for Baby's formula equipment. Even if you're nursing, you'll want to reserve a place for the food mill and such.

    Can't spare the space? Place Baby's equipment on a plastic utility tray and keep it in a handy spot on the counter.
3. With Hubby's help, go ahead and move all poisons such as furniture polish and toilet bowl cleaner to an out-of-the-reach area.
4. Keep kitchen gadgets orderly and easy to find with drawer dividers.
5. Hang pots and pans on a pegboard (to avoid excessive stooping).
6. Make a list informing helpful relatives and your husband of the whereabouts of common utensils.
7. Stock up on food supplies. Have plenty of staples on hand and as much meat and vegetables as your freezer will hold.

8. When you start cooking again, don't forget the marvelous convenience of cooking in aluminum foil and eating off paper plates.

LIVING/DINING AREA
1. To help keep things as tidy as possible, put away all decorative ornaments.
2. Collect stray odds and ends that accumulate during the day in a large straw basket.
3. Throw an attractive cover over your sofa to protect it from spills and little visitors' feet.
4. In an out-of-way corner, set up a TV tray to hold diapers and baby supplies. It might not look chic, but it'll more than pay off in steps saved.
5. Most mothers find that a small bed or cradle kept in this part of the house is a must. Your baby will also be perfectly comfortable nestled in blankets on a pallet of quilts.

THE BATHROOM
When it comes to the family bathroom, you deserve cooperation, so be firm.

1. Insist that each family member hang his bath towel up to dry after use.
2. If your bathroom doesn't have a dirty clothes hamper, improvise with an empty laundry basket.
3. Give the sink a quick weekly scrub.

4. Use a hard soap that leaves little bathtub ring.
5. Keep blue cleanser in the toilet's water box.
6. Place several throw rugs on the floor to catch water and dust.

THE NURSERY

The baby's room will be the least of your housecleaning problems. You will, however, want to be sure that everything is in a workable arrangement. Place a table or inexpensive metal appliance cart beside the baby's bed to hold various supplies.

Magazine articles and books on child care will tell you which items are necessary for the maintenance of a newborn. To avoid clutter, you might want to cover a box with bright adhesive paper and keep your ensemble neatly within.

You may not have a chest for Baby just yet, but you'll want a substitute close by. A playpen makes a lovely temporary garment holder, or you can spread a clean bath towel on the floor near the crib and stack on it the gowns and T-shirts you'll be using during the early weeks.

OTHER ROOMS

When there are older children in the family, you may be at a loss as to what to do about their rooms. *Ignore them.* At least temporarily!

If you're going to ask your family for help during those early weeks, get it where it counts. Let your husband and any capable children aid you in the vacuuming, dusting, and mopping of the main living areas.

Don't stir up discontent by asking for too much help. Even though you love your house and take pride in keeping it clean, your house can never be a home without harmony within.

1

Illness—coping with the nasties

Baby is sick. He has a different cry, a rise in temperature, a rash, or some other unusual symptom.

When you call the doctor, you should have the following information written down on a piece of paper.

1. Baby's symptoms and how long he has had them.
2. Baby's temperature.
3. The names and amounts of any medicine you might have given on your own. (Most over-the-counter medications are *not* for children under two, so check with your doctor before administering them.)

CARING FOR A SICK BABY

Temperature. Your physician will instruct you to take your baby's temperature either in the rectum or under the armpit. A normal rectal reading is 99.6° F., one degree higher than an oral temperature reading. A normal axillary (under the arm) reading is 97.6° F., one degree lower than an oral reading. When reporting the temperature to the doctor or nurse, state the method you used (rectal or axillary) and the temperature exactly as it reads.

High fever. A baby's temperature can shoot sky high at a moment's notice. You'll want to avoid temperatures around 105° F. and higher, as convulsions may result.

Make sure that you know the proper dosage of aspirin substitute. Because of the risk of your baby contracting fatal Reye's Syndrome, doctors today are *not* recommending aspirin for children. A sponge bath of cool water is also helpful for lowering Baby's temperature.

Since fever is a sign that something is not quite right, be sure to contact your doctor.

DRESSING THE SICK BABY
Keep Baby dressed in soft, comfortable clothing for the duration of his illness: no scratchy lace or tight armholes. If diarrhea is a problem, you may want to dress Baby in a gown rather than a knitted suit with feet in it.

Do give a daily bath and change soiled garments promptly.

THE SICK BABY'S ROOM
A nursery turned infirmary should be warm and free of drafts. Buy or make a mobile to

hang over the crib, and change linens frequently.

Remove pillows and toys from the bed to protect them from becoming accidentally soiled.

Respect Baby's need for quiet, and prohibit the use of television and radio in his room. There may be occasions when you'll make him a bed in the living room, or perhaps tuck him in bed beside you, but allow Baby to rest in his own crib for as long as he wants.

FEEDING THE BABY

Sick babies are not really going to eat much, but whether your baby is completely breast-fed or well into solids, ask your doctor to be specific about his diet.

Don't be tempted to coax Baby's appetite; he'll eat when he's ready.

Remember that during infections and fever, *proteins* are used up quickly, so smaller, more frequent feedings are advised—usually a liquid, semiliquid, or soft diet.

Clear liquid diet—7-UP, clear soup such as chicken broth.
Liquid diet—cream soups, plain ice cream, fruit juices, meat broths.
Soft diet—baked potato, cream cheese and crackers, gelatin.

During Baby's diarrhea, your doctor will probably tell you to begin with liquids and gradually add solids. The intestine is irritated and needs the rest, so too little food is better than too much.

Jealousy— harnessing the lion

Jealousy is one of those predictable evils that can hurt the strongest marital relationship. But if you recognize the problem and face it together, things should go a lot smoother.

COPING WITH PARENTAL RESENTMENT
Stella Chess, physician and writer, tells us that for a parent to be jealous of his new baby is quite normal and very common. We give up a little more freedom and a little more youth and time for each child that we have. Here are some ideas to help you and your husband cope with your feelings during this time of adjustment.

COMMUNICATING WITH YOUR SPOUSE
1. Don't hide your feelings.
2. Admit to Hubby that you're jealous when he leaves for work all clean and freshly shaven.
3. Ask for help when you need it, but be specific. A generalized plea for help usually only results in an argument, while a direct request brings quick action.

4. Share your worries so that the two of you can distinguish them together. Does your figure bother you? Perhaps Hubby should encourage you by exercising alongside of you. Is it low self-esteem that's getting you down? Maybe your husband can come up with a worthwhile community project for you to become involved in.

When it comes to a jealous husband, take a look at yourself first. If you're happy and feeling well, you'll find it easy to be attentive and loving to Hubby. But if things haven't begun to work themselves out by the baby's ninth month, you may want to consider confiding in a physician or pastor. He can turn you in the right direction for help.

Ignore jealousy and resentment? Never. As proof of the ultimate harm it can do to a family, reread the story of Esau and Jacob (Gen. 27:1-41).

An old-fashioned remedy for handling the jealousy "bug":
1 oz. of recognition
2 lbs. of attention
Sprinkle with love and kiss good-bye.

K

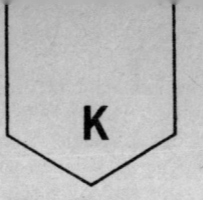

Keepsakes—
going down memory lane

Today, there are many ways to make remembering the high points of your baby's development an easier job: photographs, tape recorders, journals, and scrapbooks, to name just a few.

A scrapbook is ideal because it is inexpensive and demands little of Mom's time. Follow the directions below to create a real treasure of your own in little or no time.

MAKING A MEMORY BOOK
Materials needed:
A loose-leaf scrapbook held together with twine—available at most variety stores
About one yard of fabric. Choose from silks, dotted swiss, organza, or a delicate cotton print
Rubber cement or stapler
Scissors
Gummed hole reinforcements
Directions:
Cut the fabric two inches larger than the front of the book. Take the book apart to make handling easier. Cover the book, folding over a generous

hem. Glue or staple the hem in place. Slit the fabric above the holes in the original cover. Place gummed reinforcements around each slit.

To make your book even more precious, why not add pretty French paper, available in art supply stores, and tie it together with embroidered ribbon?

FILLING THE MEMORY BOOK

With what will you fill your keepsake book? Try for the unusual. Include such items as:

1. The sheet of paper on which you recorded your contractions during labor.
2. Hospital souvenirs—bracelets, pamphlets, schedules, doctor's written orders, etc.
3. A delivery room picture.

Make it also a book of "firsts." A few ideas:

1. Number of feedings during the first month.
2. Number of diaper changes during the first month.
3. Your first night of uninterrupted sleep.
4. Baby's first smile.
5. Baby's first coo.
6. Baby's first trip.

You'll have many questions to ask the doctor, so write these questions as well as his answers in your book. They may come in handy next time around.

One busy mother never had time to complete memory books for her three children. But while each was still a baby, she sat down and wrote him a letter, all about how wonderful it was to be his mother, and to hold him in her arms. It is a lovely idea.

L

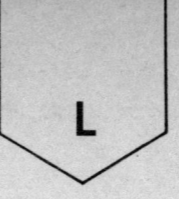

Layette—
what Baby will wear

Do be wise as you consider all the many wonderful but tempting baby products on the markets.

You might want to try one or two of each item in the list below. The first month of parenthood will determine what things you like best and need. While the number of garments you'll need for the baby will depend on your washing situation, the *style* of these garments is a matter of taste.

LAYETTE
- 6 nightgowns
- 6 shirts
- 6 sacques
- 6 kimonos
- 6 stretch suits
- 1 sweater
- 1 bonnet
- 1 pair booties
- 4 dozen diapers
- 1 bunting
- 4 plastic pants
- 2 sets of diaper pins
- 4 bibs (see instructions for making your own)
- 6 receiving blankets
- 4 blankets
- 3 lap pads
- 6 sheets
- 6 bath towels
- 6 washcloths

BIB INSTRUCTIONS

Materials needed:
1 washcloth
1 packet bias tape
Thread

Instructions for sewing:
Fold and cut the bib as indicated by pattern.
Pin bias tape to the neck opening. Sew in place.
Cut two strips of bias tape seven inches long.
Run a seam down the middle for each strip of tape.
Sew one strip on each side of the neck opening for ties.

Variations:
1. Hand-towel bibs are larger versions of the above and are especially nice for the older baby.
2. Instead of bias tape, you can close the neck opening with gripper snaps or a Velcro fastener.
3. Decorate your bibs with appliqués, lace, and embroidery.

M

Mothering—the gentle art

Which is more important, the quantity of time spent with a child or the quality of this time? Actually, both are important! To get a better picture of how they are related, try doing the following exercise.

Make a list of all the things you have to do for your child and another list of all the things you would like to do for him. Your list might look something like this:

THINGS I HAVE TO DO FOR MY CHILD
feed; bathe; diaper; care for when ill; provide clothing, toys, proper medical care.

THINGS I'D LIKE TO DO FOR MY CHILD
provide him with a comfortable atmosphere; give him good memories; give him the ability to handle stress; give him the ability to make decisions; give him a sense of honesty and sincerity; give him love and the ability to love back.

Now try it for yourself.

THINGS I HAVE TO DO FOR MY CHILD
_____
_____
_____

THINGS I'D LIKE TO DO FOR MY CHILD
_____
_____
_____
_____

Would it surprise you to learn that the wonderful gifts in the second list quite often come about as an end result of those mundane chores in the first list?

While you're performing the functional duties of motherhood, Baby is being immersed in you, the person. He's taking in your smile, your voice, your scent, your happiness or unhappiness. And although he's got a long way to go, he's slowly grasping your values and your outlook on life. So put quality into the everyday business of living; it's more important than we sometimes realize.

One smart mother made arrangements with her church's mothers'-day-out program for her children to take turns attending. This way each of her two children had one day every other week when Mom was all his.

The older your child becomes, the more avenues you'll have to explore. For now, it's probably safe to say that as long as you're smiling, kissing, touching, and complimenting the baby as often as you can, you're on the right track.

Your main goal as a high-quality mother is to let your child know that he has added joy and happiness to your life.

SPECIAL HINTS ON MOTHERING

1. Make Baby's bath more than a cleanliness routine. Purchase a book on infant swimming and help him become acquainted with the water.
2. Utilize your backpack to hold Baby during household chores. Being a real part of your world leaves a little one so satisfied.
3. Talk to your baby as you feed, diaper, and tend to his needs.
4. Stop in the middle of your housework to pat his little head.
5. Encourage the use of new skills such as grasping, standing, and pulling up whenever the baby is in your lap.
6. Make sure that the baby is always placed in as interesting surroundings as possible.
7. Provide colorful picture books and the best of music.

Natural Ways—
childbirth and nursing

While there are many good books dealing with childbirth and nursing, let's look at some information to guide you initially.

PREPARED CHILDBIRTH
What is prepared childbirth?
Prepared childbirth is training for the physical and mental control of a normal labor and delivery.

What are the advantages of prepared childbirth?
The most commonly noted advantages of prepared childbirth are these:

a. The mother goes into labor with an understanding of the birth process and the ability to cooperate with her body as it goes through the various stages of labor.

b. The mother's muscles have been prepared to work effectively during labor and delivery.

c. Although analgesics are sometimes used, anesthesia is not routinely used within a normal prepared childbirth experience.

The absence of drugs means a safer delivery for the baby.

d. During a prepared childbirth, the father becomes more than a helpless bystander. He is, in fact, the pillar of strength behind it all.

OPERATIVE CHILDBIRTH

A cesarean section (c-section), although considered by experts to be a simple operation, is still major abdominal surgery. The decision to do it requires the best of medical judgment—it's never an elective on the mother's part.

One of the most common reasons for performing a c-section is *cephalopelvic disproportion,* which simply means that the mother's bony pelvis is too small for an average-size baby to be delivered vaginally. This situation can also include a mother whose pelvis is average in size but whose baby is large.

Other reasons for this type of surgery are *placenta previa,* a condition in which the placenta is attached low in the cervix region rather than high up on the interior wall of the uterus; *premature separation of the placenta from the uterus; the breech position of a baby;* and *uterine inertia,* the term used to describe unusually weak contractions of the uterus.

Sometimes it's necessary for the doctor to perform an emergency c-section. This may happen when the pelvic disproportion is questionable, and the decision for a c-section can't be made without a trial of labor; or when there is any other reason to believe that to allow labor to continue would endanger the life of the baby.

After surgery, it might take a while for your appetite, urination, and bowel movements to return to normal. But before you know it, the usual three- to seven-day hospital stay will be over.

NURSING

Once your baby has entered the world, he will have to eat. Chemists and physicians now tell us that today's formula is *almost* as good for Baby as breast milk. So, what will it be? You or the bottle?

Breast-feeding has several advantages:

1. *Breast-feeding means fewer illnesses and allergies for Baby.*
2. *Breast-feeding is a whole way of mothering.* It's referred to as the "third and completing phase of the maternity cycle"—pregnancy, birth, then nursing.
3. *Breast-feeding is easier on the mother than bottle-feeding.* The special bond created between nursing mothers and their infants is probably one of the best known emotional advantages of breast-feeding.

Midnight feedings and colicky babies may tire the nursing mother, but they don't seem to leave her with the burned-out feelings commonly found among bottle-feeding mothers.

What causes the physical and spiritual

ties between a breast-feeding mother and her infant?

Experts tell us that it is probably due to a physiological factor, for the release of the hormone, *prolactin,* during lactation seems to contribute to the motherly instinct.

Also, both the baby and the mother have something that the other one needs. Baby needs his mother's milk, and Mother needs the physical relief that comes when Baby takes her milk. Such give-and-take is a natural part of a relationship of love.

4. *Breast milk is readily available.*
5. *Breast-feeding fits so easily and naturally into family life.* For instance, Mom can do anything from reading with a younger child to enjoying dinner with Hubby—all the while feeding her baby.

And as for going out, what could be easier than toting along a breast-fed infant? A couple of spare diapers and your own good milk are all you need to keep your baby happy.

6. *Nursing mothers often regain their pre-pregnancy figure quickly.* During and after each feeding, the hormone *oxytocin* causes the uterus to contract and actually return to its normal size faster than it would if the mother didn't nurse. Even those extra pounds accumulated during pregnancy present few problems because making milk burns up calories more pleasantly than any diet.

7. *Last, but not least, is the simple pleasure derived from nursing.* This aspect of breast-feeding is not easily understood by anyone who has not nursed; yet it is freely admitted to by those who have. Breast-feeding is not like a sexual release, but it is very much a sensual experience.

   Women will often speak of having a "physical high" while nursing their babies. One woman summed it up when she said, "God thinks of everything!" Exactly. If this pleasure were not an intended part of nursing, our Maker wouldn't have provided it; so why not accept the gift and enjoy it?

GUIDELINES FOR SUCCESSFUL NURSING

1. Somewhere around the sixth month of your pregnancy, locate a nursing league. La Leche League International, Inc., which offers support and encouragement to any woman who wants to nurse her baby, is the best known.
2. Read, read, read. Some outstanding books on breast-feeding are these:
    The Womanly Art of Breast-feeding—La Leche League International
    Nursing Your Baby—Karen Pryor
    The Tender Gift: Breast-feeding—Dana Raphael
    Abreast of the Times—R. M. Applebaum, M.D.
3. Arrange for some kind of household help, not just for those trying postpartum days, but for the duration of your nursing experience. Weekly cleaning help may be out of the question, but a thorough "once a month" job can keep your house and your morale in good condition.

4. Begin streamlining your life. Gardening, sewing, meetings, and extensive cooking can wait. Your body will set the limits; so when you're tired, rest.
5. Understand and be prepared for the emotions and special problems of a nursing mother. Preoccupation with Baby and a decreased sex drive are two common complaints, but there are others equally as frustrating. Accept these changes with the knowledge that things will return to normal when you wean the baby.
6. Learn to enjoy nursing from the beginning of motherhood. Perhaps you can make it a habit to stop whatever you're doing at least twice a day and sit down with a cup of tea or juice or milk while Baby nurses. This is a lovely chance to relax, particularly if you have other small children.

Overweight—
what goes on must come off

Nature never intended for pregnancy to result in obesity. If you don't believe it, take a look at the sleek lines of a mother horse—or any animal for that matter.

HOW TO PREVENT EXTRA POUNDS
Probably the best way to insure yourself against excessive weight gain after pregnancy is to stay within the recommended weight boundary set by your doctor *during* pregnancy. Women who work hard to establish sensible eating habits during this time are likely to eat wisely for the rest of their lives.

Curbing an expectant mom's appetite isn't the easiest task, though, and you may have to work overtime just to stay one step ahead. Have some healthful snacks:

1. Keep peeled cucumber slices and carrot sticks in the refrigerator.
2. Place a bowl of fresh fruit on the coffee table for late-night television snacks.

3. Stock up on a wide variety of vegetable and fruit juices.

Learn to estimate the caloric value of foods and how to use these calories most effectively. For instance, a banana spread with a tablespoon of peanut butter is about two hundred calories less than a chocolate bar, but much more filling and nutritious.

Your six-week checkup will probably find you almost back to your prepregnancy weight, plus five or six pounds. A nursing mother will likely lose these extra pounds during the first few months of mothering, but if you are bottle-feeding or weaning a baby and still on the hefty side, now's the time to get that weight off.

Mopping the kitchen floor may feel like hard work, but burns up only 5.3 calories per minute!

To find out how many calories you may eat each day in order to maintain your present weight, multiply your weight by 15. You'll more than likely discover that you can enjoy a normal, but moderate diet. You can also regulate your diet with exercise.

The important thing is to eat a well-balanced, nourishing diet. When you do, you'll discover that you eat only when you're hungry, crave fewer sweets, and know when to stop. Anyone who's in on these secrets should surely be slim for life.

HEALTHFUL EXERCISES
1. *Walking* is pleasantly relaxing, requires no partner, and involves no high fees.
2. After the initial investment, *biking* claims many of these same advantages.
3. *Tennis* is terrific if you can really play. But if you spend a lot of time standing, you'd best not count it as serious exercise.

P

*Pacifiers—
solving the dilemma*

WHY USE A PACIFIER?

There are a lot of reasons for using the pacifier—most of them with your infant's best interests in mind.

1. *It helps quiet a baby.* A baby who uses the pacifier to get over bouts of fretfulness will usually outgrow his desire for it as he outgrows the colic (around three or four months) or irritability.
2. *It helps satisfy a baby's need for extra sucking.* If your infant seems continuously hungry but spits up profusely after meals, he may simply be overeating to meet his sucking needs.

    Check with your physician to rule out illness, and then offer the pacifier; it may be just what Baby's been looking for.

    A good trick for a nursing mother with sore nipples: When both breasts have been emptied, allow baby to finish his sucking on a pacifier until your nipples are in better condition.

3. *It is less likely than the thumb to push teeth out.* This holds true for the special orthodontic-type pacifiers.

COMPLAINTS AGAINST THE PACIFIERS
1. *It can become a substitute for the mother.* When Baby cries, what he really wants may be *you* and what you as a mother have to offer—whether it's a feeding or a warm hug.

    The nursing mother should be particularly careful not to use the pacifier too much. It can sometimes satisfy a baby's sucking needs so well that he fails to nurse long enough at the breast, and a decrease in Mom's milk supply results.
2. *It sometimes demands more work on your part than it's worth.* If you find yourself getting up throughout the night to replace a crying baby's pacifier, you might want to take the pacifier away and pat Baby on his back instead.
3. *Baby may become so attached to it that he simply won't give it up.*

On the other hand, when a three month old starts spitting the pacifier out, it's time for Mom to put it away. Some mothers gradually ease the pacifier out of the picture by hiding it when Baby's not showing much interest.

Q

Quiet Time—moments for your Baby and you

Probably the first prayer your child will hear is a tearful, and somewhat emotional, thanksgiving for his safe delivery. But even if you choose to keep those thoughts between just you and God, the weeks ahead will provide ample opportunity for praying for your little one.

> Those that seek me early shall find me (Prov. 8:17b).

If you fail to teach your child anything else, don't neglect the area of prayer. For knowing how to talk with God is one of the most valuable gifts that can be handed down to a youngster.

Many adults think that the only suitable prayer for a child is the memorized prayer. But being able to talk to God from your heart is really what it's all about. You're trying to teach your child to use prayer as a tool for living so that someday he can move his own mountains.

SAMPLE PRAYERS FOR CHILDREN
Thank you, God, for loving us. Amen.

Dear Lord, thank you for Daddy (Mommy), and help him (her) to have a good day. Amen.

Dear Heavenly Father, we enjoyed the sun today. Please give us another pretty day tomorrow. Amen.

As Baby gets older, you'll want to talk about things that pertain to his life. Thank God for a happy outing. Or after a particularly trying day, ask him to give you both a better tomorrow. Bedtime prayers are especially adaptable to these simple conversations with God.

Sometimes a mother starts off with good intentions of praying with her infant, but as soon as life becomes hectic, prayer is the first thing to go. Don't let that happen. Find time to pray during feedings, snack times, walks, cleaning times.

BIBLE READING
Bible reading can be harder to pursue than finding time for prayer. It helps if you have a special spot to store your Bible and can go to it every day.

To get you started, here are some interesting stories of biblical mothers.

Read about:
Sarah's blessing—Genesis 21:1-8
Rebekah's twins—Genesis 25:19-34
The mother of Moses—Exodus 2:1-10
Hannah's family—1 Samuel 1–2:21

Motherly love—1 Kings 3:16-27
A mother's miracle—2 Kings 4:8-37
Elisabeth's baby—Luke 1:5-80
The birth of Christ—Luke 2
A mother's request—Matthew 20:20-23
Mothers who loved Jesus—Mark 10:13-16
Christ's compassion for a mother—Luke 7:11-15

R

Romance— restoring the sparkle

It takes longer than six weeks after the birth of a baby for a marriage to return to normal. Those first few weeks are spent in celebration and recuperation, the next few in learning how to care for your baby, and somewhere between twelve and twenty-eight weeks are spent in simply trying to keep up with Baby's demands.

No wonder that our husbands become second-class citizens, practically overnight. A good marriage is like a strong sapling—it can certainly take a little bending without causing too much harm. It is, however, pretty safe to say that a woman who is tuned-in to life will recognize her husband's silent pleas for attention.

LOVE STRATEGIES
1. Of course, you're taking care of your appearance—dressing neatly, smelling good, and exercising faithfully. Now, choose a usually ordinary night like

Monday and greet your husband at the door in a hostess gown complete with earrings and necklace.
2. Prepare a midnight feast to be eaten off a tray in your bedroom
3. Go out—just the two of you—for a few hours. Even a nursing mother can leave her little one to a sitter for two hours.
4. On your absolutely worst day, set a candle on the table and *voila!*—a candlelight dinner.
5. Surprise your husband with a love box full of paper clips and rubber bands. Directions: Paste magazine pictures of lovers, sunsets, children, etc., on a small cardboard box. Shellac for a shiny finish.
6. Turn your bedroom into a private retreat. One set of pretty sheets, a scented candle, and an FM radio do wonders for a romantic interlude.
7. Put Hubby first once in a while. For instance, when the baby is crying for simple attention and you're in the middle of pouring your husband's coffee, let the baby cry until you've taken care of your man.
8. If you find yourself thinking of your husband as nursemaid relief, think twice. To assure yourself the energy you'll need to be a loving wife, take naps during the day and never use all of your strength on housekeeping.
9. Have a romantic picnic for two. All you need is a loaf of French bread, a block

of cheese, olives, and a thermos of spice tea.
10. Praise your husband for his fathering skills, for his eagerness to help, and for his lovemaking. Everyone appreciates knowing his worth.

Finally, one of the nicest things about romance is that with just a tiny bit of encouragement, a small spark can grow into a huge fire.

S

Schedules— getting yours in order

TEN WAYS TO MANAGE YOUR TIME
Believe it or not, you can organize your day without falling prey to a rigid hourly time schedule.

1. *Decide what your priorities are.* These are the things that we *must* do in order to be at peace with ourselves. Strive to do these each day *before* attempting the extras.
2. *Do your most dreaded chore when your energy is at a high.*
3. *Make a weekly list of the things you want to accomplish.*
4. *Hire people—professionals or teenagers —to do strenuous jobs such as window cleaning and lawn mowing.*
5. *Hire people to do those things—sewing, hair coloring—that require an expert's touch.*
6. *Subscribe to a good family-oriented magazine to keep up with new products, etc.*

7. *Reevaluate how you're presently spending your time.*
8. *Find out what things, if any, are draining you of energy, such as care of fancy appliances. Streamline your life.*
9. *Have simple daily goals* to give you a great sense of accomplishment. Use the Daily Goal Chart.
10. *Ask for God's guidelines in planning your activities.*

DAILY GOAL CHART
Things I must do: _____

Things I should do, but don't have to: _____

Things I like to do: _____

Things I hate to do: _____

Now, using the Weekly Activities Chart, divide each day of the week into three segments—morning, afternoon, and evening. Place those things which you must do in their workable time slot.

WEEKLY ACTIVITIES CHART

Day	Morning	Afternoon	Evening

Last of all, check to make sure that you aren't tied down to dreary obligations that don't really matter. Because in addition to caring for your family, there should be time for rest, fun, and meditation in every day.

Most important, when the day is over and you've done all that you can humanly manage, don't try to do more. Be proud of what you've accomplished.

A Mother's Prayer

Dear Lord,

As I start each day, help me to rearrange my priorities so that I am receptive to your love and guidance and am willing to place these things first. Amen.

Traveling— have Baby, will bundle

In spite of transportation marvels, traveling with Baby is not easy. Here are some ideas to make your trips more enjoyable.

PLANNING AHEAD
Now that Baby's here, there will be no more meandering holiday jaunts. You should know well in advance how you will travel and where you will be going. Determine what kind of preparations must be made for Baby's food.

1. *Milk*. Mother's milk is always sanitary, always warm, and always there. But for a fairly reasonable price, even the bottle-feeding mother can claim convenience. Today's prepared formulas come in pre-measured bottles that require no refrigeration and no preheating, and can be thrown away after use.

   Of course, if you'll only be traveling for twenty-four hours or less, there's no need to go to this expense. You can prepare your formula at home and pack it in an ice chest or an insulated bag.

Use your own bottles lined with disposable nurser bags for easy cleanup. If Baby insists upon warm milk, stop at a roadside cafe and ask the waitress to heat the bottle for you. Or if you're traveling by plane, a flight attendant will gladly help out.

2. *Solids.* When Baby starts to eat solids, those commercial foods that you might shun at home are heaven-sent. Select foods that are well-liked and familiar. If Baby must be fed from your plate, offer him nongreasy, warm foods.

Avoid cold meats, fish, eggs, milk puddings, and cream-filled pastries, as these foods are among those most likely to cause illness.

Carrying a thermos of distilled water and peeling your own fruit are two other safety measures you'll want to consider.

MINI-SURVIVAL KIT
There's something comforting about nibbling, no matter what our age or how far from home we may go. Instead of giving Baby candy sticks, round hard candy, and peanuts that might be easily choked on, try packing a generous portion of toasted whole-wheat bread slices. This treat is much easier for Baby to digest and much easier for you to clean up.

PACKING

Even when you're packing tight for the rest of the family, Baby needs two bags—a suitcase and a tote bag. I call the suitcase *Baby's overnight bag* because this is usually the one I don't have access to until we're in our motel room. Into this bag go all the things I would normally need for a given time period at home—only twice as much of everything.

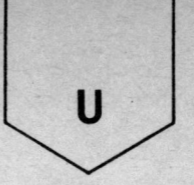

Unity—
plugging for each other

God believes in the family. At no time has he ever condoned the destruction of a family through divorce, infidelity, or homosexuality. The family is one of man's most treasured gifts from God.

ENRICHING FAMILY LIFE
Strengthening family ties offers a lot of fun and challenge:

1. Begin by instituting the custom of weekend family outings. (No baby-sitters for Saturday afternoons, please.)
2. Have a time of daily devotionals with each other. Perhaps an evening prayer with Mother and Dad is all that the very young baby will enjoy, but the length of devotional time can grow as he does.
3. "Roughhouse" together. Pillow fights and jumping on a bed can be surprisingly fun for an old stick-in-the-mud. Just be sure that such activities stay within reasonable bounds.

4. Select and watch a good television program together. Then take time to discuss it.

MOTHER'S ROLE

Mothers have a special role in building the family. They should be gentle and yet unyielding to unruly ways. Encourage everyone to respect other members. Never allow family members to speak unfavorably about each other. Teach even the youngest member of the family to understand the needs of other members.

Last of all, accept the responsibility and authority granted to you as a mother and use it wisely. For the love that God gave you and your husband is from this point on eternal and everlasting.

V

Vaccinations—keeping up with Baby's health

Breast-feeding and a balanced diet can go a long way toward protecting your baby against illness, but they should never be thought of as substitutes for recommended immunizations. This is crucial to remember since polio, diphtheria, whooping cough, tetanus, measles, and mumps are still very much alive and just as dangerous as ever.

Don't depend upon the doctor or the nurse to keep you posted on which immunizations your child should have and when. If you ask, they will gladly supply you with a schedule and perhaps even a record card for keeping track of the dates on which the inoculations were given.

Tape the schedule where you can keep your eye on it during Baby's first year. Then place it in your favorite child-care book for easy reference.

MEDICAL RECORD

Vaccinations   *Date*   *Notes*

Diphtheria
Whooping cough
Tetanus
Polio
Smallpox
Measles
Mumps
Rubella
Boosters

Tests

Illnesses

W

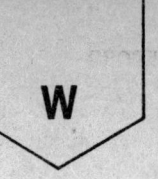

Working—pros and cons

To work outside the home or not? You'd think by now we mothers would have resolved this question. But we haven't. Those of us who are working are still feeling guilty about leaving the nest, and those of us staying at home are still remorseful about that money we're not earning.

Like so many other difficult decisions, when it comes to choosing between a career and full-time mothering, you have to make up your own mind, and you have to be aware that what's right for the lady next door may not be at all suitable for you.

Two Truths to Consider
1. Children do not ask to be born.
2. Children have a right to expect both a mother and a home.

Most mothers admit that it would be best to stay at home with their baby, but where does that leave those who have to add to the family income? Ideally, when a mother has to earn money, both parents should strive to find a way of supplementing the income without causing her to forfeit her desire to stay at home, at least part of the time.

It might be comforting to some women to know that combining a career with homemaking is, in fact, biblical. King Lemuel describes such a situation to his son as he talks of the perfect wife.

> *She finds wool and flax and busily spins it.*
> *She buys imported foods, brought by ship from distant ports. . . .*
> *She goes out to inspect a field, and buys it; with her own hands she plants a vineyard.*
> *She is energetic, a hard worker, and watches for bargains.*
> *She works far into the night.*
> *She sews for the poor, and generously gives to the needy.*
> *She has no fear of winter for her household, for she has made warm clothes for all of them. . . .*
> *When she speaks, her words are wise, and kindness is the rule for everything she says.*
> *She watches carefully all that goes on throughout her household, and is never lazy.*
> *Her children stand and bless her; so does her husband (Prov. 31, TLB).*

No one could accuse this woman of sitting at home twiddling her thumbs. But notice that although she did indeed take part in monetary matters, she also took care of her family.

If you can manage your career and your home life in a similar way, more power to you. A lot of women would like your secret. In the meantime, the rest of us had better turn to a part-time job.

---

7 Ways to Work Part Time
- Baby-sitting
- Sewing
- Baking
- Manuscript typing
- Door-to-door sales
- Hostessing children's parties
- Telephone sales

X

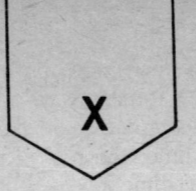

X's of Family Fun— the secret's out

> To every thing there is a season, and a time to every purpose under the heaven:.... A time to weep, and a time to laugh; a time to mourn, and a time to dance (Eccles. 3:1, 4).

Celebrations are important. Not only are they just plain fun, they're miraculous in reviving low spirits. Now that you're a family, celebrating will take on a different shape from those old twosome days. For example, instead of celebrating your engagement date, you'll turn all of Baby's "firsts" into grand occasions.

A YEAR OF FUN
Holidays will also provide hours of fun with your family. Here is a list of some major ones around which to plan your good times. Take a moment now to jot down ideas to make the days special.

- New Year's Day (January 1) _____

- Valentine's Day (February 14) _____

- April Fool's Day (April 1) _____

- Easter (March or April, depending on the moon's phase) _____

- Mother's Day (Second Sunday in May) _____

- Children's Day (June 12) _____

- Father's Day (Third Sunday in June) _____

- Independence Day (July 4) _____

- Labor Day (First Monday in September) _____

- Thanksgiving (Fourth Thursday in November) _____

- Christmas (December 25) _____

Y

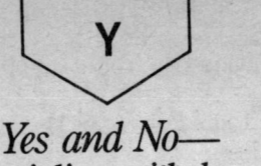

Yes and No— discipline with love

First of all, strike the notion that discipline is punishment. Think of it as teaching and training—training that's necessary in order to live happily and safely in our society.

Schoolteachers tell us that their best teaching results come when they give guidance and place control on their pupils, but then stand aside so that learning can take place. This is in essence what parents are doing when they set limits and take a stand on issues that children can't handle.

Children need parental guidance. They can't cope with complete freedom, although even an eighteen-month-old baby will do his best to convince you he's capable.

Please remember that you can't spoil a baby. To allow Baby to cry from hunger, wetness, or boredom isn't discipline—it's cruelty.

FOUR TECHNIQUES FOR MAKING BABY MIND

Spankings? Certainly not for anyone under the age of two!

Distraction is a handy device in baby discipline. Nature makes this form of discipline instinctive up to a point. Baby grabs the diaper pin without even thinking; Mom exchanges the pin for powder. Apply the same techniques with your older baby.

Rewards are another way to teach the young child or toddler who is beginning to learn right from wrong. Baby plays quietly during nap time, even though he thinks he's getting too big for rest periods, and you reward him with a small surprise and the remark, "Because you were so good."

Of course, *teaching by example* is also an effective discipline method. And it's easy because you simply treat your baby with the same courtesy and respect that you'll expect from him someday. Knock on his bedroom door before entering, and use "please" and "excuse me" in your speech.

But you'll probably find the *reinforcement of praise and love* to be your most effective disciplining tool. Praise your baby for goodness even when it's bound to be "accidental" on his part.

EVEN IF YOU FAIL

There'll be times when you miss the mark completely. Don't be afraid to apologize. Your apology will help your child regain his dignity and his faith in you. He may be only a baby, but he's still a person.

> Train up a child in the way he should go: and when he is old, he will not depart from it (Prov. 22:6).

Z

Zzzzz—
sounds with meaning

Experts tell us that mothers have a natural gift for teaching speech. And it all begins with that first coo. Mother smiles with delight at this tiny sound and coos back in imitation. Baby thinks this is a lovely game and an even lovelier way to win a twinkle from Mom's eye.

Soon he says a sound that resembles a word in the tiniest way, and it becomes a household word. "Give him his ba," Mom orders Dad. And bingo! Baby has discovered the power of communication.

Now he must learn the secrets of this wonderful thing called talking. He takes time for watching others make those all-important sounds, noticing the shape of their mouths, the placement of their tongues, even the muscles in their necks.

Practice, practice, practice. Baby does that on any sound he can happen upon as he babbles. When we hear these musical sounds early in the morning, we say he's playing quietly in his bed—actually, he's working, and diligently, too.

Left solely in the hands of nature, babies do an amazing job of learning to talk. But when parents help, things go so much faster, and learning becomes a fun game for everyone involved.

TEN COMMANDMENTS FOR TEACHING SPEECH

1. *Speak clearly and slowly at all times.* This gives the baby a chance to catch and isolate certain sounds. When you're talking directly to him, try exaggerating the shape of your mouth once in a while, and remember to put end consonants on words that end with the letters *t, d,* etc.
2. *Face your baby when talking to him.* He wants and needs to see the body language that accompanies speech. In fact, you'll find that unless the young baby sees your face, your words sometimes carry no meaning.
3. *Never push your baby in his speaking efforts.* While it's probably true that early speech is a sign of intelligence, it shouldn't be used as conclusive evidence one way or the other. Einstein, by the way, didn't talk until he was three years old.
4. *Repeat words when talking to the baby.* Repetition is an old but proven teaching method that works as well in talking as in anything else.
5. *Give all objects a name.* For instance,

when you're powdering the baby, say the word *powder* aloud and hold the can where he can see it.
6. *Listen to your baby's language—foreign as it may be.* Let your face show that what he says is important. If you don't give him this courtesy, he's likely to give up with a "what's the use" attitude. Besides, the sooner the baby learns that listening is part of communication, the easier your life will be.
7. *Never leave your baby in the care of someone who speaks poorly.* Your child will imitate the speech of whomever he spends the most time with. Thus, if for some reason you must spend a great deal of time away from home, use the utmost care in selecting a baby-sitter.
8. *Let your child watch educational television shows.* Children's shows such as *Sesame Street, Mr. Rodgers,* and *Electric Company* fascinate even the very young baby and are great vocabulary builders.
9. *Keep your speech free of profanity.*
10. *Speak in a pleasant, friendly manner.* Sarcasm, nagging, and complaining will produce a whiny, irritable child, and it certainly won't help the home atmosphere either.

TALKING GAMES

1. *Experiment with sounds as you play with your baby.* Copy the baby's sounds and then make up a new sound for him to

copy. You may discover that he doesn't even attempt this sound until days later. (Perhaps he's practicing in private.)
2. *When the baby is around nine months old, make him an alphabet sound book*. You can draw the letter and illustrate it with a picture that explains the sound. Example: "Sammy the snake makes *Ssss* sounds in the grass." Try reading to Baby during mealtime.
3. *Name each object as you dress the baby.* Example: "Now let's put on your sock." (Hold up sock.)
4. *Play the question game.* Example: "Where is Baby's shoe?" (Hold up shoe.) "Here is Baby's shoe."
5. *Hang a mirror knee level to you on a wall in the baby's room.* Sitting in front of it, show Baby how to watch himself make different sounds.

Other Books for New Mothers

Baby and Child Care by Dr. Benjamin Spock (New York: Pocket Books, 1971).

Better Homes & Gardens New Baby Book by Better Homes & Gardens Editors (New York: Bantam Books, 1980).

Building a Christian Home by Henry R. Brandt and Homer E. Gowdy (Wheaton, IL: Victor Books, 1978).

The Christian Family by Larry Christenson (Minneapolis: Bethany Fellowship, 1970).

Happy Mother, Happy Child by Nancy Moore Thurmond (Wheaton, IL: Tyndale House Publishers, 1982).

How To Raise Good Kids by Barbara Cook (Minneapolis: Bethany Fellowship, 1978).

The Idea Book for Mothers by Pat Hershey Owen (Wheaton, IL: Tyndale House Publishers, 1981).

The Mother's Almanac by Marguerite Kelly and Elia S. Parsons (New York: Doubleday & Co., 1975).

The Spiritual Needs of Children by Judith Allen Shelly (Downers Grove, IL: InterVarsity Press, 1982).

About the Author
JAYNE GARRISON is the author of *The ABC's of Christian Mothering* and *The Christian Working Mother's Handbook* (Tyndale House). She lives in Arlington, Texas, with her husband, Olie, and their two daughters, Heather and Alexandra.